You and Your Hair

The Ultimate Healthy Hair Masterclass
For
Afro-Textured Hair

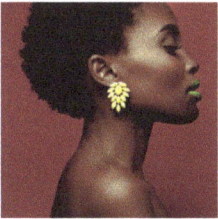

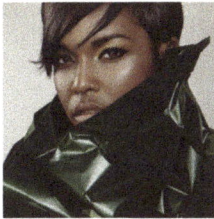

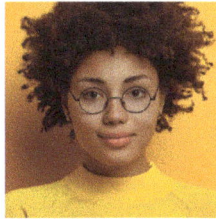

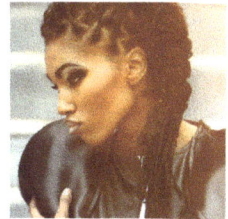

**Celebrating and respecting
our individual hair as equally
unique and beautiful**

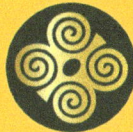

Health and Beauty

You and Your Hair

First Printed in United Kingdom 2020

Published by Conscious Dreams Publishing
www.consciousdreamspublishing.com

Edited by Lee Dickinson
www.wordwisewebltd.com

ISBN: 978-1-913674-08-3

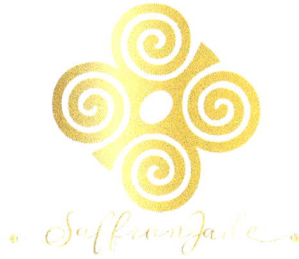

You and Your Hair

*You are enough, You are beautiful, You are unique,
You are loved*

Positive health and well-being for
Afro-textured hair
A holistic approach to healthy haircare:
Making a positive difference to people's lives through
education, knowledge and empowerment

SARAH ROBERTS

About the Author

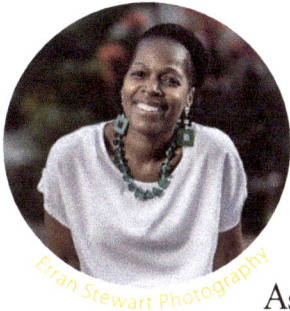

Erran Stewart Photography

S arah Roberts is a healthy hair consultant, educator, and passionate advocate for the overall health and well-being of Afro-textured hair. Sarah has a BA Hons in Applied Social Studies and is an Associate Member of 'The Association of Registered Trichologist'. Over the last 22 years, she has engaged with women and children to promote a positive sense of self-identity, emotional well-being, strength and resilience in the areas of positive parenting, healthy relationships and the development of self for personal growth and progression.

Over the last ten years, Sarah has consulted and educated women, men, children and young people about the science and special care needs of Afro-textured hair, supporting them to develop an individual healthy haircare regimen to achieve healthy hair and longer lengths.

Sarah loves to engage and communicate with people in the areas of healthy hair, education, culture and identity. She has a passion for children and advocates for their overall well-being and happiness. Sarah is passionate about her family and enjoys creating lasting memories by spending quality time together.

She likes to think of herself as an everyday athlete and enjoys keeping physically fit through regular exercise and engages in meditation for mental and spiritual wellness.

www.saffronjade.co.uk

you@saffronjade.co.uk

Instagram: Saffron_jade19

Contents

Introduction

As the founder of Saffron Jade, I would like to present to you the ultimate healthy haircare masterclass for Afro-textured hair, celebrating and respecting our individual hair as equally unique and beautiful.

Our hair is our biggest accessory, it's our crowning glory, part of our unique identity. Our hair has a voice and unique characteristics. Its special make-up allows us to create a vision of beauty and creative art, tells a visual picture of culture, identity, fun, sophistication, style and finesse.

Saffron Jade takes a holistic approach to the overall health and well-being of women, men and children and the care of Afro-textured hair. The main aim is to educate, empower, motivate and inspire women, men, children and young people to understand the science of our Afro-textured hair and the care it needs to be healthy, strong, grow long and have a healthy individual shine. This will promote self-love, a positive sense of identity, self-acceptance and positive self-esteem in regard to our cultural heritage, history and ethnic identity.

I am passionate about making a positive difference to people's lives, through education, knowledge and empowerment. My engagement with women and children over the last 20 years has enabled me to promote a positive sense of self-identity, emotional well-being, strength and resilience in women's lives, in areas of positive parenting, healthy relationships and the development of self for personal growth and progression. Over the last ten years, I have pursued my passion to promote and share my knowledge of healthy hair within the black and mixed heritage community on the beauty and special care needs of Afro-textured hair, whether natural, relaxed or locs. My love and passion for natural hair is well known by my friends and family, but I fully respect a woman's individual right to choose how she wears her hair.

My mission, passion and goal, is to inspire, motivate, educate and guide the black and mixed heritage community to reflect on the relationship they have with their own hair, taking the time to assess whether they have a heathy haircare regimen which allows them to see the true beauty of their individual hair.

Together we can begin to create a collective understanding and give a new meaning to 'good' and 'bad' hair. 'Good' hair represents healthy hair that has a balance of moisture and protein, which is what our hair needs to be strong, soft, have an individual shine and reach long lengths, if this is our preference. 'Bad' hair represents, unhealthy hair that is dry and brittle, due to a lack of moisture and protein balance.

This handbook is designed to guide you through a journey of information and knowledge for you to begin to develop a positive relationship with your hair and become the expert at what your hair needs for its optimum health and well-being. Some of the information overlaps and will therefore be repeated to some extent. However, this reinforces essential information and learning which I think is both helpful and necessary for some readers. The information within the book will cover:

- A basic understanding of the structure of hair and the unique difference of Afro-textured hair

- A basic understanding about how a healthy lifestyle helps promote healthy hair

- The importance of a healthy scalp for healthy hair growth

- Understanding the unique characteristics of your individual hair, so you can adopt a healthy haircare regimen, tailored to your hair's individual needs

- Understanding the difference between hair growth and keeping the growth

- The root causes of common hair loss and hair damage for Afro-textured hair

- Understanding the importance of feeding your hair essential healthy nutrients through healthy product selection

- Developing your personal healthy haircare regimen to achieve healthy hair and longer lengths.

Our Hair

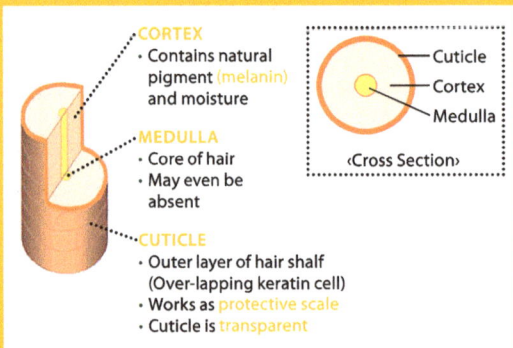

CORTEX
- Contains natural pigment (melanin) and moisture

MEDULLA
- Core of hair
- May even be absent

CUTICLE
- Outer layer of hair shaft (Over-lapping keratin cell)
- Works as protective scale
- Cuticle is transparent

Cuticle
Cortex
Medulla

‹Cross Section›

Our hair is an attachment to our skin, namely our scalp which produces a natural oil called sebum to condition our hair.

Our hair is made up of two separate structures:

1. The follicle, which exists below the skin and is the living part of the hair.

2. The hair shaft, which is the hair that we see.

This part of our hair is dead and is made up of three layers of keratin which is a form of protein:

Our Hair

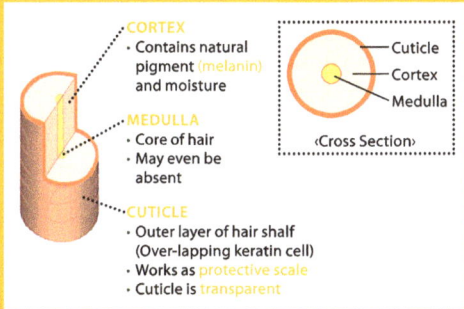

CORTEX
· Contains natural pigment (melanin) and moisture

MEDULLA
· Core of hair
· May even be absent

CUTICLE
· Outer layer of hair shaft (Over-lapping keratin cell)
· Works as protective scale
· Cuticle is transparent

Cuticle
Cortex
Medulla

‹Cross Section›

MEDULLA
Is the inner layer, not present in all hair types (E.G: people with fine hair types).

CORTEX
Is the middle layer. It makes up the majority of the hair shaft. This is where most of the hair is made up in regards to its strength and where the moisture is.

CUTICLE
Is the outer layer, which is formed by tightly packed scales in an overlapping structure that resemble roof shingles.

Our Hair

Afro-textured hair differs from other ethnicity's in the basic shape of the hair fibre, as it has **bends**, **curls** and **twists**.

Each of these:

- *Bends*
- *Curls*
- *Twist*

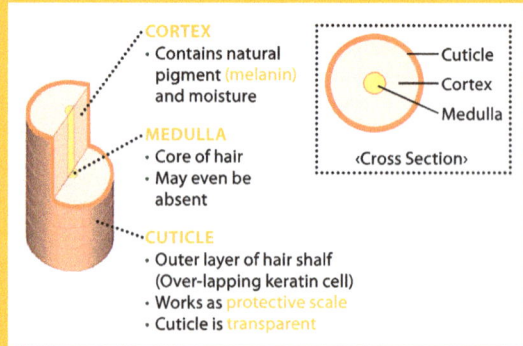

CORTEX
- Contains natural pigment (melanin) and moisture

MEDULLA
- Core of hair
- May even be absent

CUTICLE
- Outer layer of hair shaft (Over-lapping keratin cell)
- Works as protective scale
- Cuticle is transparent

Cuticle
Cortex
Medulla

‹Cross Section›

represent a breaking point regardless of if your hair is natural or relaxed. Making it the most fragile and vulnerable of all hair types.

Think of
our hair
as
A FIBRE

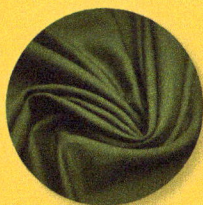

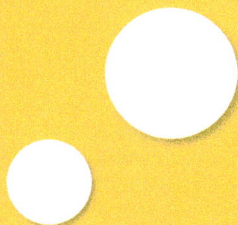

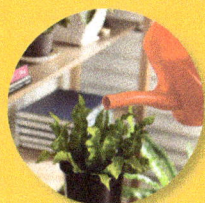

- As delicate as silk, unique to each of us, with its own individual identity and character

- Similar to a plant, our hair thrives on water, as it needs moisture to keep it from breaking

- Chemically altered hair (relaxers) is even more fragile than natural hair, and needs even more care and attention

CHAPTER 1

Our Hair

*Celebrating and Respecting Our Individual Hair
as Equally Unique and Beautiful*

It's important for us to acknowledge a lot of the information about the care and nurture of Afro-textured hair has been lost to many of us for a long time. So, open your mind to this rediscovered information as new learning for us and get ready to discover the true beauty of your hair, whilst getting to know and understand your hair more intimately.

The two parts of cells that make up our hair are the root that sits within the hair follicle and the hair shaft, also known as the hair fibre. Once our hair grows out of our scalp, it is essentially dead. This means it is unable to maintain any level of health and well-being, without you looking after your hair, giving it the love, care and nurture that it needs to grow healthy, long and keep strong.

Our hair fibre is made up of mostly protein and has three layers: **medulla**, **cortex** and **cuticle**. These layers all play a role in keeping our hair healthy, with the main two parts being the cortex and cuticle. Depending on the thickness of your hair, which relates to the texture of your hair, some people do not have the medulla, which is part of the internal structure of the hair fibre, as explained in the coming pages.

The **medulla** is the innermost layer of the hair fibre and is generally only found in thicker hair types. This is part of the internal hair structure.

The **cortex** is also part of the internal hair structure and makes up the greatest percentage of the hair fibre. This part of the hair is where the strength and elasticity originate. This is also where the moisture is captured, and it determines the hair colour.

The **cuticle** is the outer layer of the hair, the external structure. Its purpose is to shield and protect the cortex of our hair. It's essentially made up like the slates of a roof on a house. The layers overlap to protect the cortex and keep it from getting damaged. The healthy appearance of hair generally depends on the condition of the cuticle. Tattered and damaged cuticles often result in the hair looking dull. When cuticles are damaged and raised instead of lying flat, like those on a roof, it results in greater friction between the cuticles.

Chemical treatments, such as relaxers, hair-colouring and harsh shampoos that strip the hair of essential moisture, all play a significant part in wearing away the hair's protective cuticle layers. Also, rough handling of the hair and using unhealthy combs and brushes aggressively also damage the outer cuticle. This daily wear and tear of the hair is known as 'weathering'.

Afro-textured hair types are unique and beautiful. However, they are the most fragile of all hair types due to the basic shape of the hair fibre, which has bends, curls, twists, coils and kinks. Each of these represents a breaking point, which is why the hair is 'fragile' and as delicate as a silk fibre. When Afro-textured hair is chemically straightened, the natural bends, curls and twists still exist and continue to represent a breaking point, which makes relaxed hair more fragile than when it is in a natural state. This means the care and nurture it requires is important to understand in order to keep the hair healthy and strong and from breaking constantly.

What is the function of Sebum and its relationship to our hair's health and well-being?

The main function of sebum, the natural oils produced by the scalp, is to lubricate and condition our scalp and hair. However, our beautiful curls, twists, coils, kinks and bends make it difficult for our natural sebum to travel down and coat our hair fibre, which is why our hair is essentially dry and requires regular moisture to address this challenge. In this sense, water is not our enemy, but our hair's best friend. Think of our hair as a beautiful plant. Plants cannot survive without water. When plants do not receive enough water, the leaves become dry and brittle and the plant eventually dies. This is the same process for our hair. Our bodies need water to feed our cells and our hair needs to receive regular hydration and a good level of moisture, so it does not become dry, brittle and dull. The ultimate method to ensure that our hair receives hydration is by washing and conditioning our hair regularly, by adopting a consistent healthy hair care regimen. This will stop our hair from breaking off at the same rate that it is growing. Your goal is to preserve your hair fibres from being damaged and protected from the day-to-day manipulation of styling, washing, combing and the environment.

As we go through the masterclass, you will learn more about the various ways we add moisture and protein to our hair fibres to keep them healthy and strong by adopting a healthy haircare regimen of:

- Cleansing/washing
- Conditioning
- Deep conditioning treatments
- Moisture sprays
- Using products that have water as a key ingredient.

Adopting a Healthy Lifestyle for Healthy Hair

Understanding the importance of having a healthy balance of

'Mind, Body and Spiritual Well-being:

helps us to be conscious about ensuring that we are constantly working towards this balance, as they work as a system;

when one element is out of balance, it impacts the others.

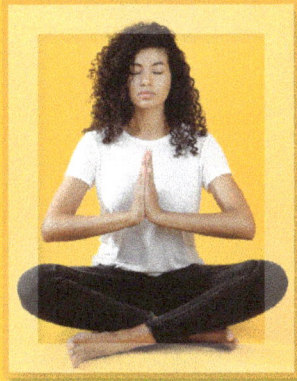

MENTAL & EMOTIONAL WELL-BEING

PHYSICAL HEALTH & NUTRITION

SPIRITUAL WELL-BEING

Mental & Emotional Well-being

A balance of happiness, laughter, fun, relaxation, feeling of security, and positive self-esteem

- Impacts on the care and attention we give to ourselves, which includes our hair.

- Impact on our eating habits, as our emotional state can often dictate our choices.

- Impacts on our motivation to want to make positive changes for our overall health, which includes our hair.

- Too much stress can seriously affect our hair growth.

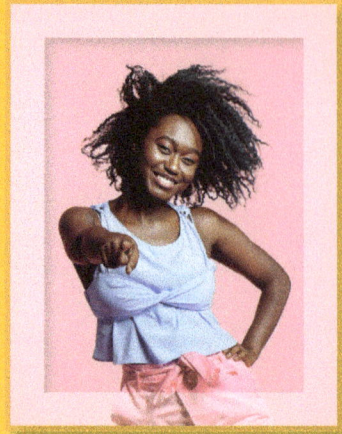

Physical Health & Nutrition

A good nutritional diet, foods consisting of protein and essential foods, with vitamins and minerals that the body needs to help your hair grow and keep it strong and healthy.

Ill health and medication can impact the health of your hair.

A good exercise regimen will support healthy hair growth.

Changes in hormones can have an impact on the health of your hair.

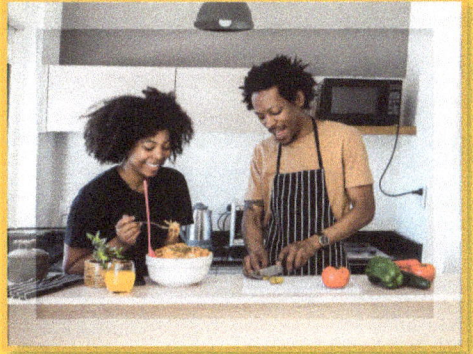

Spiritual Well-being

A readiness for enhanced spiritual well-being is defined as an "ability to experience and integrate meaning and purpose in life through a person's connectedness with self, others, art, music, literature, nature, or a power greater than oneself." This supports a positive sense of 'self: to promote self-confidence, self-love and self-belief.

- Negative attitudes and feelings about our hair can result in neglect, not giving enough care, time and attention.

- Love and acceptance of our beautiful hair is key for us, our children and younger generation.

- Our words are powerful. It is important for us to move away from 'good hair', 'bad hair', 'difficult hair' and feelings of our hair being ugly, in comparison to other hair types.

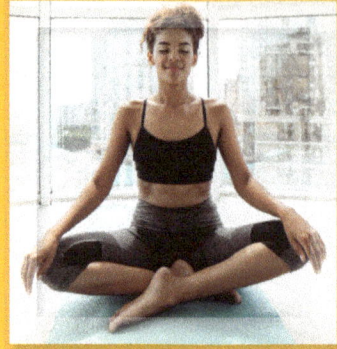

CHAPTER 2

Adopting a Healthy Lifestyle for Healthy Hair

✦

You are enough, You are beautiful, You are unique, You are loved

Our hair is our biggest accessory and plays an important part in representing us to the outside world daily. Afro-textured hair has been misunderstood regarding its beautiful structure and the care and nurture it requires to look and feel its best. In this sense, it's important for our hair to look its best, which means it needs to be healthy. However, the health of our hair is also dependent on our overall health and well-being, such as our physical health, including the food we eat to nourish our bodies. Mental and emotional health also impacts our behaviour, and motivation and spiritual wellness provides a sense of purpose, fulfilment and contentment.

Being conscious of the importance of having a healthy balance of mind, body and spiritual well-being helps us in several ways:

1. We can develop a greater understanding of how all three elements work as an overall system, thus when one element is out of balance, it impacts the others.

2. We can prioritise these three areas as a continued approach to a healthy lifestyle and keep striving to proactively maintain a healthy balance.

3. It helps us to reflect and recognise what areas we might need to work on and/or what support we need to achieve greater balance.

Our Scalp

The birthplace of our hair

Understanding the importance of a healthy scalp to grow healthy hair

Our scalp and hair need to be thought of separately.

The scalp is skin that needs to be treated the way we treat our facial skin-regular cleansing.

Kept clean and free from dirt and build-up of products that can block the pores.

CHAPTER 3

Our Scalp

The Birthplace of Our Hair

When we think about the health of our hair, it's important for us to think of our scalp in two ways:

1. Separate from our hair

2. The birthplace of our hair

The scalp is essentially an extension of the face. It needs to be kept clean and remain moist to ensure it's a healthy environment for healthy hair. Our natural sebum adds essential moisture to the scalp, although it is recognised that scalp dryness is a common complaint within the black community, and this is said to be related to a genetic lack of sebum production at the scalp level.

A healthy scalp regimen includes:

- No heavy oils or greases to block the hair follicle – only use 100% natural oils or ingredients to moisten the scalp if required

- Cleanse the scalp weekly or fortnightly to remove bacteria, dirt, build-up of sebum and products. Use a shampoo that nourishes the scalp with healthy ingredients. The routine normally helps women to eliminate problems with dandruff.

- Massage the scalp – this can be done whilst washing to stimulate blood flow to cells for greater hair growth

- Be careful not to scratch or damage the scalp with sharp nails, combs

- Ensure hairstyles, weaves, braids, clips are not too tight, adding tension to the scalp

- **Eat healthy** – A well-balanced diet will help supply the skin of the scalp with the raw materials necessary to produce new, healthy cells.

Notes

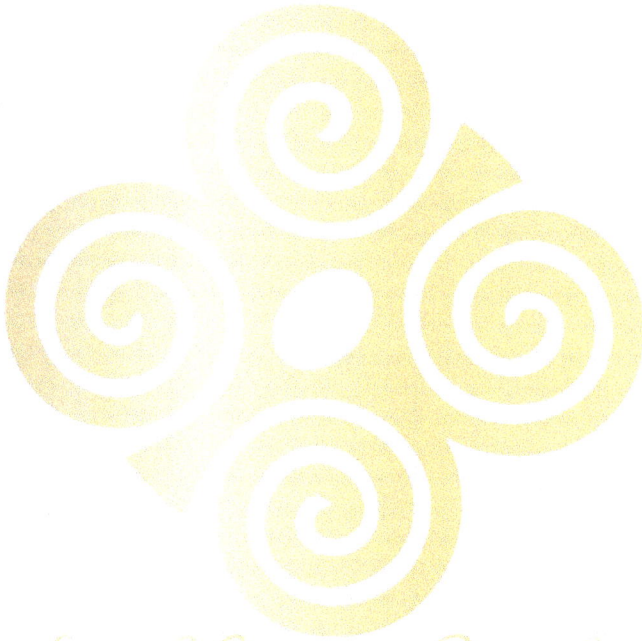

'You' and Your Hair

Getting to know the characteristics of your hair

What do you need to know and understand about your hair?

CURL PATTERN

TEXTURE

POROSITY

ELASTICITY

DENSITY

CHAPTER 4

You and Your Hair

Getting to Know the Characteristics of Your Hair

This section of the handbook is very important, as it's essentially about you developing a positive relationship with your hair, which means taking the time to get to know the characteristics of your hair whilst adopting a holistic approach to healthy haircare.

Healthy haircare should always begin at home, with you being the expert on your own hair. It's part of self-care and needs to be passed down to our younger generation so we can change the script for generations to come. For some of you, this development will be totally new and, like any new relationship, there are various stages I have experienced and seen other women go through from my healthy hair consultations over the years that can be related to the five stages of a relationship. It's important for us to acknowledge that not everyone goes through all five stages. However, I think it's useful to recognise the stages, so you can know the emotions and behaviours are very 'normal' and you can get through them.

Stage One: Fantasy Phase
(also known as the Honeymoon Stage)

This is the beginning of your hair exploration. You are motivated to begin a regimen and try new methods and products. You are having lots of fun with the idea of understanding the different characteristics of your hair. You begin with a positive attitude and mindset, looking forward to improvements in the health of your hair, its length and feel. You are looking forward to trying all the fantastic hairstyles you have seen on Instagram and other social media platforms.

Stage Two: Reality Stage

Reality starts to take over. You begin to realise that understanding the characteristics of your hair is not as simple as everyone makes out, as other factors related to health, age and environment can affect our hair. You might be experiencing some frustration at still not being able to figure out what works well for your hair, including the moisture and protein balance your hair needs. The fantasy is wearing off. Some of you might want to give up on your healthy hair journey. These feelings are perfectly normal. However, if you just relax, with patience and consistency, you will begin to develop an understanding of the characteristics of your hair. This will allow you to manage and provide the care it requires, so it looks and feels its best.

Stage Three: Disappointment

What began as reality setting in during Stage Two can turn to disappointment in Stage Three. You might be disappointed at your lack of progress, as we often want to see quick results, and have unrealistic goals. We sometimes want fantastic results without putting in the effort to warrant them.

You also might be comparing your hair with others. This is also normal but remember the unique characteristics of your hair is what makes you a unique individual. Getting to know and understand your own hair takes time. Our hair is unique to each of us and will respond in its own way to different methods and products. In this sense, trial and error is part of the journey. This is the stage where you need to love and respect your individual hair as unique and beautiful. When Afro-textured hair is healthy, whether natural, relaxed or locs, it looks worlds apart from unhealthy hair. Unhealthy Afro-texture hair often looks dull, feels dry and brittle, will break easily, experiencing breakage in different parts of the hair.

Stage Four: Stability

If you can push through the challenges of Stage Three, you will begin to experience feeling more confident in understanding your hair allowing you to enjoy the journey more. You may have more patience and not set too many unrealistic goals. Your consistent care will enable you to see improved health in areas of:

- Hair fibres being thicker, due to increased moisture from a consistent cleansing regimen, allowing the correct balance of moisture within the cortex of the hair fibre

- Hair being softer with more elasticity and stronger due to the correct balance of moisture and protein conditioners being used

- Hair looking hydrated and having a natural shine.

You begin to accept the unique beauty of your individual hair and can admire other curls and women, but respect and celebrate your own. This will allow you to feel more connected to your own beautiful hair and help you understand that collectively our hair is equally beautiful and unique.

Stage Five: Commitment

In the world of relationships between people, we are told very few couples make it this far. However, I am more than confident you will reach this stage, and well done to all who already have. This commitment to your hair is your commitment to yourself. You are deserving of investing in yourself. You and your hair are truly a team, respecting its challenges and the overall beauty and possibilities.

We will revisit what commitment looks like at the end of this masterclass when looking at your individual healthy haircare regimen.

Notes

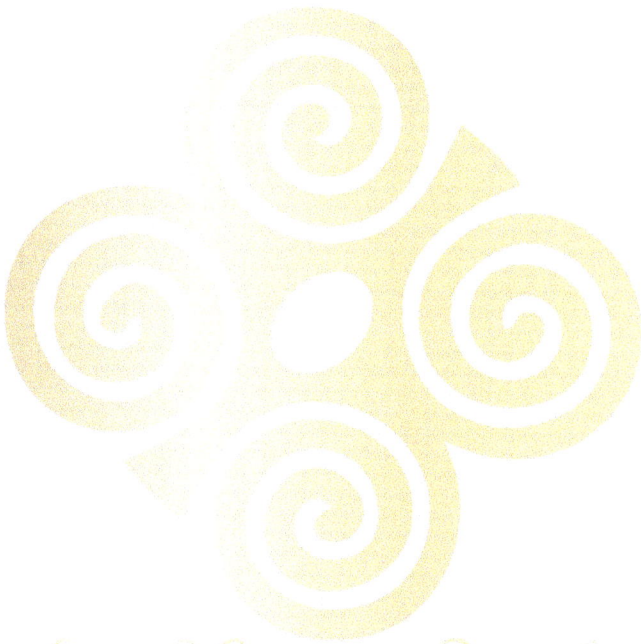

Curl Pattern

✿ **Loose Curls**

✿ **Curly**

✿ **Coily**

✿ **Tighter Curls & Coils**

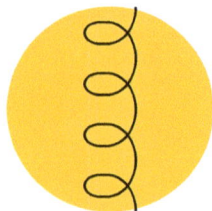

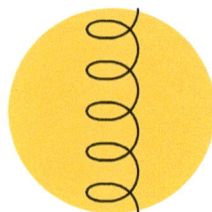

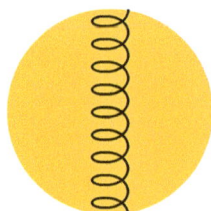

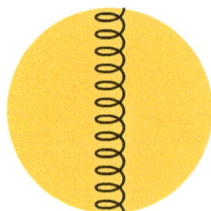

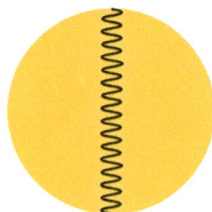

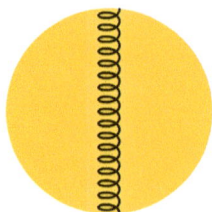

You and Your Hair

Understanding Your Curl Pattern.
Celebrating and Respecting Our Individual Hair
as Equally Unique and Beautiful

Hair type and curl pattern both describe the shape of your hair as well as how hair naturally grows, such as straight, wavy or curly hair types. Each head is unique, like our fingerprints. Afro-textured hair is naturally curly, and the shape or pattern of our curls is determined by the shape of our hair follicle. The more oval its shape, the curlier the hair will be. Heat, chemicals, damage and a lack of moisture presented in the cortex of the hair can alter how your curl pattern presents itself. In this context, lots of us are walking around not even knowing we have a beautiful curl pattern. We know from our African ancestry and from the women and men living in different parts of Africa today that Afro-textured hair is very diverse, and our curl pattern can range from:

- Loose curls
- Curly
- Coily curl
- Tighter curls and coils.

Most of us will have a combination of different curl patterns, with one or two different patterns being the most dominant. The tighter the curls, linked to more bends and curls, the more fragile the hair is, as remember each bend, kink, coil represents a potential breakage point. Moisture is a key factor to ensure hair is soft and able to stretch and be manipulated without breaking.

Understanding our curl pattern, along with the other characteristics such as texture and porosity, helps us to understand how to care for it properly, which will be directly linked to these characteristics. Some Afro-textured hair types are drier than others, due to the unique curl pattern, and will therefore need more pampering and effort to keep it moisturised. Remember, all curls are equally beautiful, whether loose, curly or coily, including tighter curls and coils.

Notes

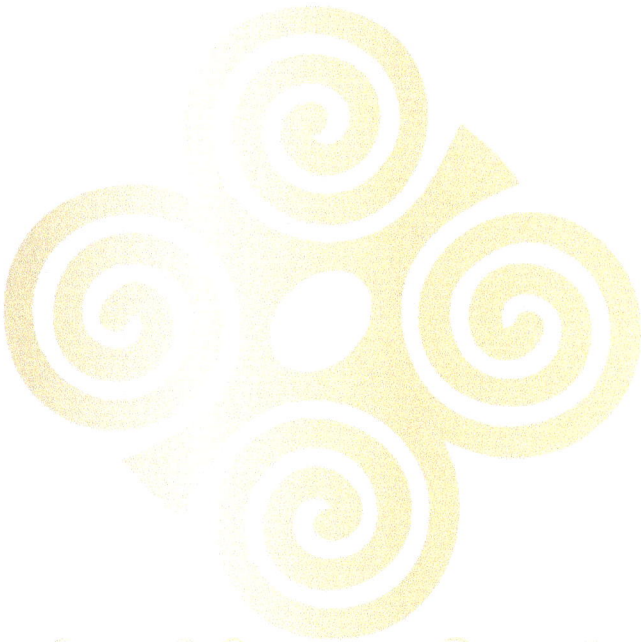

The 'Texture' of Your Hair Fibre

❖ **FINE** – thinner than a thread

❖ **MEDIUM** – same thickness as a thread

❖ **THICK** – larger than a thread

You and Your Hair

Understanding Your Hair Texture

Hair texture describes the circumference of your hair. There are essentially three different hair texture types – fine, medium and thick. Each hair texture type has its own traits that set it apart from other hair textures and influence the care or treatment it may need from you, as part of your overall healthy haircare regimen.

Some hair textures will fall between fine to medium and medium to thick. The best way to help determine our individual hair texture is to compare it with a normal piece of sewing thread. Using a strand of your hair:

1. If your hair is thinner than the thread, your hair texture is fine.

2. If your hair is equal to the thread, your hair texture is medium texture.

3. If your hair is thicker than the thread, the texture of your hair is thick.

Fine hair is the most fragile hair texture, as it is not as durable as medium or thicker hair strands. Each individual hair is thin and generally only has two hair layers: cortex and cuticle. If you have this hair texture, you will need to be extra careful as to how you manage your hair. Don't use combs, brushes and heat that can easily damage your hair strands. If you have relaxed hair, remember your hair is more fragile and therefore needs extra care to keep it strong and healthy. If you have locs, be careful not to get them retwisted too often, and not too tight.

Medium hair is what most people are reported to have. It is thicker than fine hair. The individual hairs have the same two hair layers that fine hair has but may also have the third one – the medulla. Medium hair can keep hairstyles better, looks thicker and is more resistant to breaking, but still fragile by the nature of the hair structure.

Thick hair, which is often referred to as coarse hair, has all three hair layers: cortex, cuticle and medulla. The reference to the hair being coarse is not a reference to the feel of the hair, but the size of the hair strand. This can be very confusing, so I prefer to simply talk about hair textures as being fine, medium and thick. Thick hair gives the impression of a fuller head of hair, and it can hold a hairstyle well. If your hair texture is thick, your hair is more tolerant to heat, styling products, hair dye and breakage than fine or medium hair. However, it is still fragile by the nature of the hair structure.

Understanding your texture will help in re-evaluating your overall hair regimen and what is best for your hair's health and preserving the strands. Don't forget to pay extra special attention to protecting the ends of your hair, as this is the oldest part, and more vulnerable to breakage.

Notes

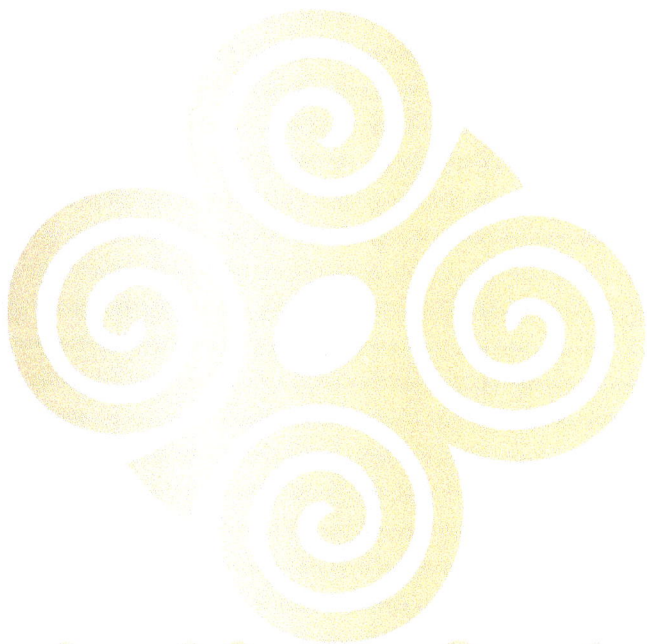

Porosity

PO-RO-SI-TY =
your hair's ability, or inability to absorb
water, products or chemicals into the cortex.

LOW – doesn't really absorb moisture

MEDIUM – retains moisture well

HIGH – absorbs water quickly,
but loses moisture just as quickly

You and Your Hair

Understanding Your Porosity

HAIR POROSITY TYPES

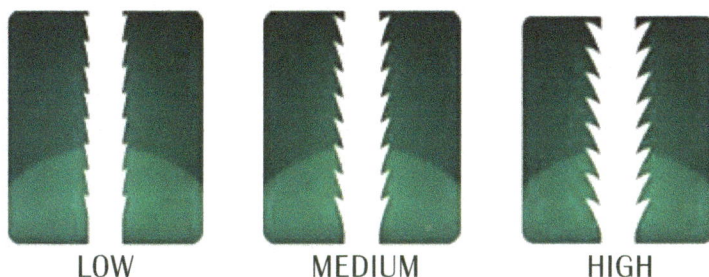

LOW	MEDIUM	HIGH

Hair porosity can be confusing, but once you understand the concept, it becomes easy. Porosity is your hair's ability or inability to absorb moisture into the hair's cortex (and chemicals, including hair dye) and is broken down into three categories:

1. **Low** – Means your cuticles are a little tight and generally resistant to receiving water and moisture. Your hair will also experience difficulties absorbing products. Low-porosity hair requires a lot more moisturising and benefits from ingredients such as shea butter, jojoba oil and coconut oil. It also benefits from products which attract and hold moisture in your hair. Choose lighter, liquid-based treatments to ensure your hair is not heavily loaded with products. You will most likely need to moisturise your hair daily.

2. **Medium** – Hair with medium porosity generally requires less maintenance due to the cuticle layer being looser, which then allows just the right amount of moisture to enter and prevents too much moisture escaping.

3. **High** – Is where the hair cuticle is highly raised or even damaged (can be genetics), which means it quickly absorbs moisture. High-porosity hair can also lose moisture quickly and will need products that can seal in the moisture to protect the hair from becoming dry and brittle.

   High-porosity hair is often damaged by harsh chemicals, dye high heat, or harsh shampoos that strip the hair. Hair can become tangled very easily as the raised cuticles catch on each other, resulting in friction between the hair strands. Light protein treatments will be required to support the damaged cuticles.

This characteristic of your hair is very important to know and understand, as you can then ensure your individual healthy haircare regimen is one that ensures your hair has a healthy level of moisture and protein balance.

Testing your hair's porosity:

- Place clean hair strands in a glass of water and wait a minute or two.

- If the hair floats and stays at the top of the water, this is an indication you have low-porosity hair

- If your hair sinks to the bottom of the glass, this is an indication you have high-porosity hair

- If your hair stays somewhere in the middle, this is an indication you have medium porosity.

Notes

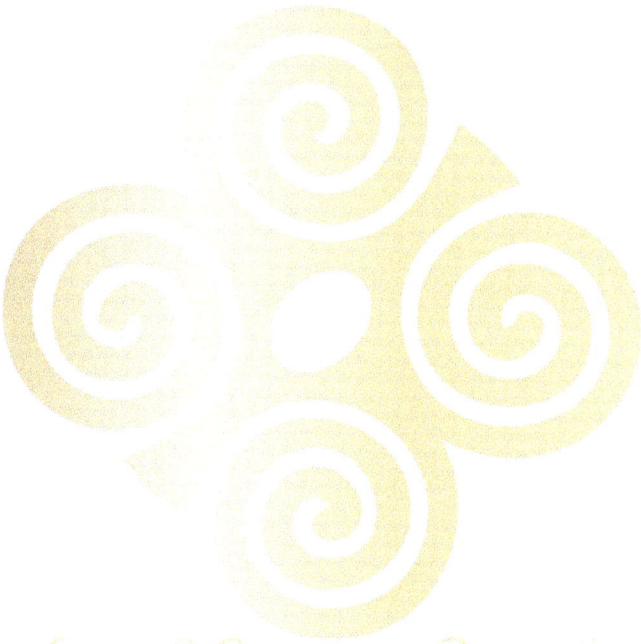

Elasticity
&
Shrinkage

The beautiful character which allows us
to have puffs, volume, creativity with our hair.

Indication of its health and vitality.

Healthy hair can stretch and return
to its original state without
breaking.

You and Your Hair

Elasticity and Shrinkage

The unique and special character of our hair, known as 'shrinkage', allows us to present our hair as a creative aspect of our identity and culture. Afro-textured hair can shrink by up to half its size. This shrinkage is normal and is also linked to our hair's character of elasticity, helping us to identify and measure its health. When Afro-textured hair is healthy, it can stretch and return to its original length many times over without breaking.

How much elasticity does your hair have?

Being aware of your hair's elasticity is an important part of understanding its health. You can check this as part of your healthy hair care regimen when your hair is wet. Simply choose a few hair strands from different parts of your head. Stretch the hair strands and then see if they return to their original length when released. Strands that return to their original length when stretched are healthy. Hair that breaks or does not bounce back is an indication that it needs to be strengthened by using a light to medium protein treatment.

How thick are your strands?

One major factor that influences hair's elasticity is the texture of our hair strands – fine strands are weaker than medium or thick strands, which can withstand more force. The part of each hair strand that contributes most to elasticity is the interior hair fibre, or cortex, as noted earlier in section one of the masterclasses.

Why you must maintain your hair's protein structure.

In the beginning of the masterclass, we spoke about the importance of keeping our hair hydrated by ensuring it's washed and conditioned regularly to keep it healthy. We also spoke about preserving our hair's internal structure (the cortex), which holds the strength of the elasticity. Damage to the internal hair structure can happen when the outside cuticle layer is broken. To limit this kind of damage:

- Avoid the use of excessive heat on your hair where possible

- Always use a heat protector for the cuticle and cortex when using heat

- Use protein treatments as part of a healthy haircare regimen, to restore damaged hair and keep it strong and resilient to everyday manipulation.

Notes

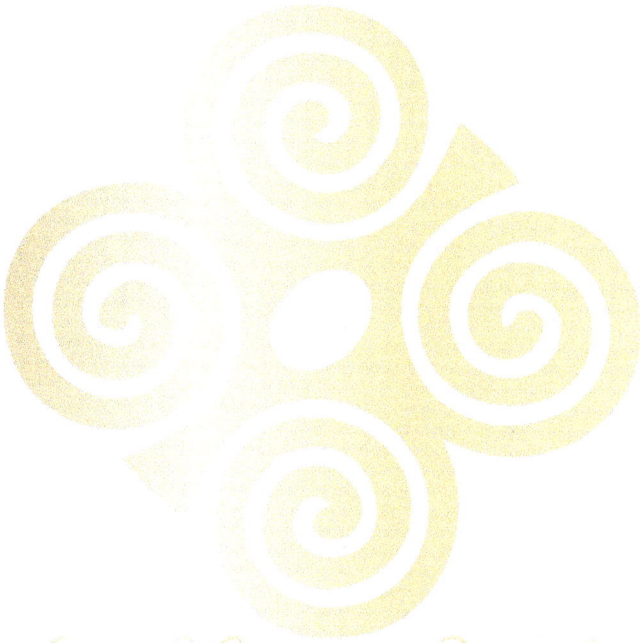

Density

The amount of hair fibres on your head per square inch

You and Your Hair

Understanding Density.
Celebrating and Respecting Our Individual Hair
as Equally Unique and Beautiful

Like all other characteristics of your hair, understanding your density will help you to choose the right products and hairstyles to show your hair at its best. When we talk about hair density, we are simply referring to how many hair follicles are on your head. Some people have a lot of hair on their head and some have less. We are told the average person has about 2,200 strands of hair per square inch.

There are several ways to determine if you have low, medium or high-density hair. If your scalp is easily visible, this indicates you have low curl density. If your scalp is somewhat visible, this indicates medium curl density, and if your scalp is barely visible, you have high hair density. The texture and curl pattern of your hair will be a factor as to how your hair looks, compared with someone with the same density, making your hair unique.

Low-density hair generally requires the use of light products that will not weigh your hair down and reduce its volume if you want it to look fuller, especially if you have fine hair strands. Low-density hair also works better using clips for ponytail hairstyles, as bands highlight the low density of your hair.

Medium-density hair can generally use a variety of products and various styles to enhance your texture, but this also depends on if you have fine, medium or thick hair strands. A mousse-type product will allow for more volume, or use heavier creams and butters to give your hair more weight and hang to your curls.

High-density hair generally allows you to choose a variety of products, depending on what look and style you want. Heavy products such as gels, creams and butters will be able to hold your curls together and reduce volume, if this is what you want to achieve. A light mousse will allow you to achieve volume.

Notes

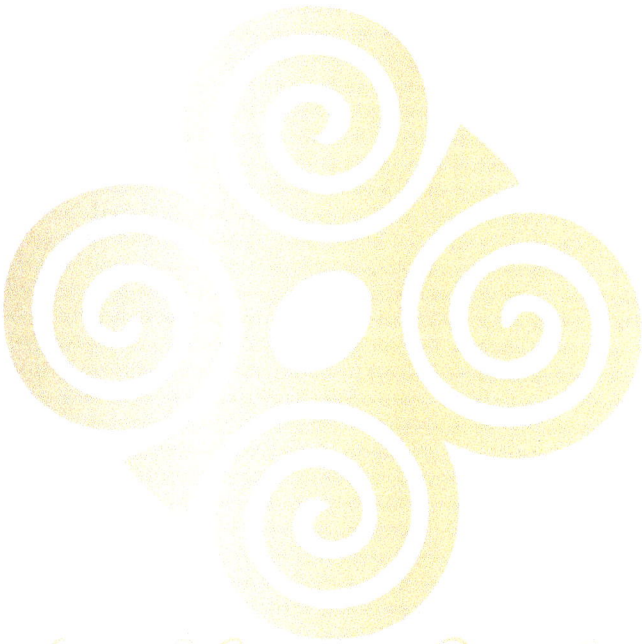

Most Popular Statements / Questions

• **My hair does not grow.**
Difference between growth and length retention.

• **My hair is very dry.**
Natural oils from our scalp is unable to travel down our curls – the need for regular wash / conditioner and moisture sprays and products.

• **How do you get those curls?**
Regular hydration and conditioning regimen.

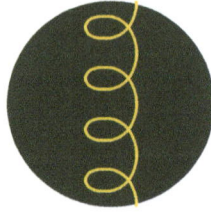

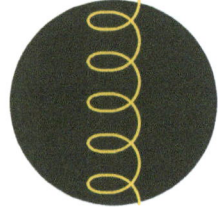

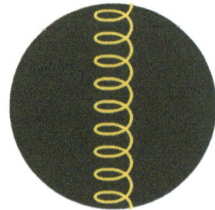

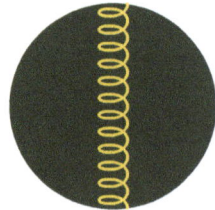

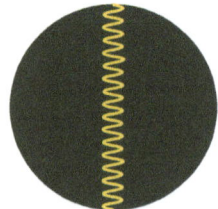

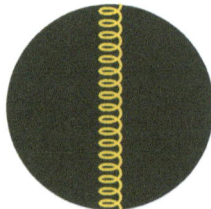

CHAPTER 5

The Three Most Popular Statements and Questions

"My Hair Does Not Grow"

How we feel about our hair can have a direct impact on how we treat it and believing it does not grow can affect the relationship you have with your hair, such as the care and attention you think it deserves. First things first – you need to believe me when I say your hair IS growing.

In looking at why it appears your hair is not growing, you need to understand the difference between hair growth and hair retention, also known as length retention.

Hair Growth: Afro-textured hair grows at an average of half an inch per month, which works out at six inches per year. As explained in Section Three of the masterclass, your scalp needs to be cleansed regularly to allow your hair to come through in its best health. Other important healthy lifestyle practices for hair growth include:

- Weekly or Fortnightly shampoo to ensure scalp is clean from product build-up, natural sebum and dirt

- Not putting heavy, unnatural products on your scalp that block your hair follicles

- Having a balanced diet and regular physical activity to feed your cells to ensure healthy hair growth

- Understanding that growth can be affected by hormone changes brought on by factors such as pregnancy, illness and menopause

- Having a balance of fun, laughter and relaxation to combat the everyday stress of daily life, which can cause serious hair loss

- Ensuring your braids, weaves or hairstyles are not too tight, which adds stress to the hair follicle and ultimately leads to bald patches and can result in permanent hair loss.

Hair Retention: Simply means adopting a healthy haircare regimen to preserve your hair strands and keep the hair that is growing from breaking off, which means you will then see growth each month.

The Three Most Popular Statements and Questions

"Why is My Hair So Dry?"

This has been talked about already within the handbook. However, it is something which comes up all the time, so I wanted it to have its own section. If you feel you have a good understanding about this aspect, simply skip this.

It's important for us to understand a lot of the information about the care and nurture that Afro-textured hair requires has been lost for many years. A reflection on our hair's history will be addressed in a book planned for later in the year.

This means that a lot of the practices we have followed (or not) have worked against what our hair needs. This has meant we have been unable to see the true beauty of our hair's overall health, look, feel and the longer lengths we can achieve, but did not believe to be possible.

One such misinformation around Afro-textured hair is that we do not need to wash our hair often and that our hair does not like water.

As already covered in Section One of the masterclass, our beautiful hair thrives on moisture, just like beautiful plants. The ways in which our hair gets essential moisture to keep it healthy and strong is from a healthy haircare regimen that is consistent with these methods and use of products:

- Washing, conditioning and deep conditioning, which will provide the ultimate moisture into the cortex of the hair fibre, ensuring it is kept hydrated until the next wash and conditioning regimen

- Regular use of Saffron Jade Leave-in Conditioning Moisture Spray between wash days will add essential moisture and hydration with organic ingredients to nourish the hair and scalp

- Hair continues to need essential moisture whilst in braids, weaves, locs and whilst wearing wigs.

The Three Most Popular Statements and Questions

"How do you get those natural curls?"

The natural hair movement, which started in America and has made its way to the UK and Europe, has resulted in many positive changes for the black and mixed heritage community. The drive on women wanting to move away from the use of chemicals resulted in a significant drop in sales of products and marketing for chemically treated hair. This resulted in the cosmetic world investing in making and marketing products researched and designed for use on natural hair. This then resulted in:

- Greater knowledge and understanding around the science of Afro-textured hair and what it needs to be healthy, whether natural or relaxed (via chemicals), and greater focus on locs as a preference for natural hair

- Greater information via Google and YouTube by women sharing their stories of using this knowledge to change the way they previously cared for their hair. The main changes related to the increased frequency of washing and conditioning, so hair is fully hydrated. This then allows your beautiful curl pattern to reveal itself, as hair was previously lacking in essential moisture, due to us not having this information and the cosmetic world not being invested in making products for our hair.

The question is, therefore, not "How do you get those curls?", but should be:

"What do I need to do, to see my naturally curly hair?"

- Adopt a healthy haircare regimen of weekly/fortnightly washing and conditioning, deep conditioning to allow water and essential healthy ingredients to fully penetrate the hair's cortex. This regimen needs to be consistent over three to six months to see significant results.

- Once your curls begin to reveal themselves, you can then use products designed to set your curls, such as gels, curling creams, curling custards and curling mousses to set these beautiful curls, showcasing the hair that was designed just for you, your ethnicity and cultural identity.

- Your curls are unable to be truly revealed if your hair is damaged, for example by heat.

Notes

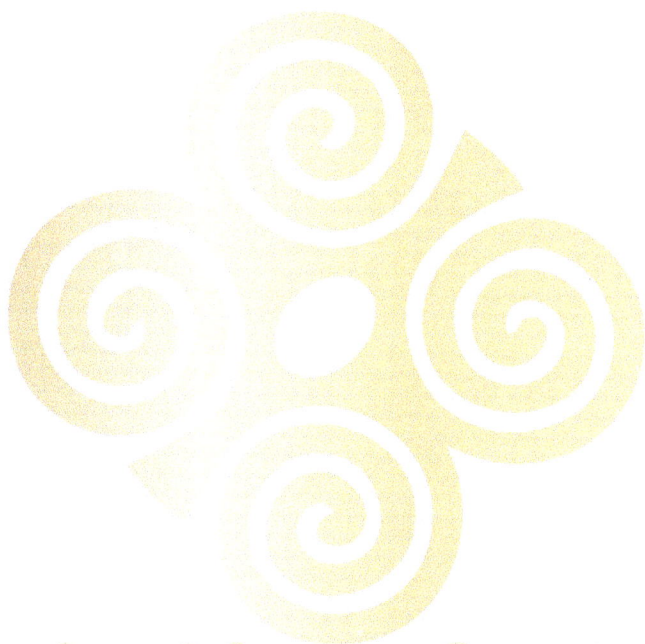

Hair Loss
&
Hair Damage

- *Stress*
- *Hormones*
- *Heat damage*
- *Tight braids / weave*

CHAPTER 6

Hair Loss and Hair Damage

Hair loss for women of any age can cause a lot of stress, with many not knowing where to turn. There are many reasons hair loss and hair becoming damaged can occur, some of which are highlighted below. However, being aware of the many causes of hair loss will help you to seek help from your GP in the first instance to rule out any internal issues that might be the root cause. This can then support you to look at various options, naturally where possible, to help your hair grow back by adopting a healthy haircare regimen and positive lifestyle changes.

1. Stress
2. Hormones – pregnancy and menopause
3. Medication
4. Genetics
5. Nutrition Deficiency
6. Heat damage
7. Illness
8. Chemicals – relaxers and hair dyes
9. Unhealthy hair practices, linked to braids, weaves, wig
10. Ignorance of healthy haircare practices
11. Harsh brushes and combs which strip the hair's cuticle

The hair loss I am going to focus on in this section relates to common problems a lot of women and young girls are experiencing, because of:

- Tight hairstyles

- Tight weaves and braids or leaving them in too long

- Locs being twisted too tight

- Unhealthy haircare practices due to a lack of knowledge about the science of Afro-textured hair and the care and nurturing our hair needs.

Alopecia is a medical term that refers to hair loss. Traction alopecia is hair loss caused by repeatedly pulling on your hair. Black women and women of mixed heritage are experiencing traction alopecia by having tight ponytails over a long time. The use of chemicals, especially over a longer period, and using heat on our hair, makes us more vulnerable to hair loss.

Early signs of alopecia might present as little bumps on your scalp that look like pimples. This is generally visible with tight braids. The hairs along the front and sides of your scalp are most often affected, as these are generally finer hair strands, so naturally more vulnerable to breaking off or coming out of the hair follicle completely. Can traction alopecia be reversed? Yes, but only if you stop wearing the tight hairstyles, such as tight braids, weaves and locs. If you continue to wear these tight hairstyles, hair loss can become permanent.

Hair damage: Damage to our hair can be caused in several ways. It can be caused from chemicals such as relaxers, which break down the hair's structure making it prone to breakage. Over a longer period, many women begin to experience (traumatic alopecia) which is caused by injury to the scalp from the constant use of chemicals. If you are experiencing traumatic alopecia, you should stop using chemicals to prevent the possibility of permanent damage to your hair follicle leading to permanent hair loss. Heat can also damage our hair and the overuse of hair straighteners as well as using a hair dryer on a high temperature can seriously damage the hair cuticles. Limit the use of heat on the hair and always use a heat protector product to protect the hair from damage.

Hair left in braid/weaves extensions for too long, without applying essential moisture: You can wash and condition your hair every two to three weeks whilst in braids, to ensure your hair is being consistently hydrated and provided with essential nutrients for its overall health. If you are only washing your hair every four weeks when you take the braids out, your hair needs to be sprayed with a moisture spray every two days. Spray to where your hair ends in the braids. Once you remove the braids, ensure you carry out a deep condition. This will also be true for weaves left in the hair for too long, without washing and conditioning the scalp and hair for its overall health. Women via YouTube channels demonstrate how to wash your hair whilst in weaves and braids.

(cosmopolitan.com/uk/beauty-hair/advice/a48958/hair-loss-reasons/)

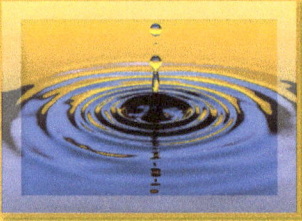

CLEANSING

MOISTURE

PROTEIN

DEEP CONDITIONER

SAFFRON JADE

CREAMS

LOC

TOOLS

The Purpose of Products for Healthy Hair and Longer Lengths

Water is the key ingredient to give our hair the ultimate moisture that it needs.

CHAPTER 7

The Purpose of Products for Healthy Hair and Longer Lengths

A Balance of Moisture and Protein

I hope, by now, you have started to understand the characteristics of your hair with the goal of preserving your hair strands, by ensuring your hair receives a healthy balance of moisture and protein. In this sense, understanding the products and how they relate to ensuring the health of your hair is vital. Products should be viewed as food for your hair, with the main purpose of providing your hair and scalp with the healthy ingredients needed for optimum health. In this sense, it's important for you to begin to understand 'healthy product selection'.

Quality haircare products, together with a healthy haircare regimen, can make a significant difference in the overall health and quality of your hair; its look, feel and overall strength. Some products contain harmful ingredients for our overall health and well-being. Your hair is unique to you and will respond differently to products, depending on the overall health of your hair strand, texture, porosity, curl pattern. Other factors include whether your hair has been chemically altered or a dye applied. Also, the products you've been using on your locs, and ensuring you don't have a build-up of them. Also consider the environment where you are living. Humidity plays a big part in the moisture balance that can be retained in your hair.

How to choose healthy products for your hair: It can be very confusing when trying to choose healthy products. A good start is to choose ones that list these ingredients as **not** being present in shampoos and conditioners due to the harmful effects on our hair, skin and body: no silicones, mineral oils, petroleum, parabens, phthalates or sulphates. It can be very challenging to find products that don't have all these harmful ingredients but use this as a guide. The more of these you see listed as **not** being present in the product, the better it is for you and your hair.

Mineral oils and petroleum: These types of ingredients are not natural or pure, so can result in your hair and scalp being blocked, causing not only skin irritation, but also preventing your hair from growing healthy and strong.

Parabens: Parabens are also known as xenoestrogens and are generally used as a preservative. They have received lots of media attention over the last few years, due to the claimed risks to our health, as they have been linked to the disruption of hormones and an increased risk of cancer. This ingredient is labelled on hair products as **propylparaben, benzylparaben.**

Phthalates: These are chemicals linked to hormone disruption and cancer. This is because, when we use products in our hair, we are absorbing the products through our scalp. These chemicals have been banned by the European Union for our safety, but remain in some products if made in other countries.

Sulphates: Sulphates are used in products to clean the hair of oil and dirt. However, they are harsh chemicals which strip Afro-textured hair of its natural oils, leaving our hair feeling dry. Our hair, as you now know, is naturally dry, due to our unique curl pattern, and needs essential moisture to keep healthy and soft and from becoming brittle and ultimately breaking. Common sulphates in products are **sodium lauryl sulphate, sodium laureth sulphate, ammonium lauryl sulphate**.

Silicones: Silicones are an unnatural substance that coats the hair, like a plastic coating, making it feel soft and smooth. Using silicones over a prolonged period can lead to a build-up on the hair, starving it of essential moisture, which leads to it becoming brittle and unhealthy.

There are a few different types of silicone, known as water-soluble silicones and non-soluble silicones. The water-soluble version is made to dissolve in water. The non-soluble silicone is unable to be removed or penetrated with water and will need the help of a clarifying shampoo. Non-soluble silicones are known as **cyclomethicone, dimethicone, methicone, amodimethicone, dimethiconol**.

Regular Cleansing / Shampoo

Allows the hair / cortex to collect essential moisture for it to remain strong and healthy — sulphate free, no silicone

Weekly / Fortnightly

The Purpose of Products
for Healthy Hair and Longer Lengths

Shampoo / Cleansing
Detangling the Hair Before Shampoo

Detangling our hair before using shampoo is essential to help with knots and tangles, which are a big factor in our hair being vulnerable to breakage. This process needs your time, focus and patience, so don't rush. You can also detangle using a natural oil as a pre-conditioner before washing, such as coconut oil, olive oil, avocado oil, jojoba or a mixture of these oils. Section your hair in four to six loose braids. Use your hands to gently remove any knots and tangles carefully, section by section, to maintain the hair's cuticle for protection of the inner part of your hair structure, namely the cortex, as discussed in section one of the masterclass.

Shampoo / Co-wash: The purpose of using shampoo / or a different method of cleansing has two functions to support the overall health of your hair.

1. For cleansing the scalp by removing dried sebum, any dandruff, environmental dust and residues of haircare products left on the scalp. This allows a healthy environment for your hair to grow and flourish.

2. In the first section of the masterclass, we talked about the cortex being the main section of our hair that

holds the moisture, elasticity and strength of our hair fibre. The function of washing our hair serves to give it the vital water that it needs to maintain a good level of hydration, and retain moisture to keep it from becoming dry and brittle, which results in the hair breaking at the same rate as it is growing.

Moisturising shampoos, especially those that are sulphate-free, will cleanse the hair gently without stripping it bare of the natural oils.

The recommended frequency of cleansing our hair and scalp is between five to ten days, depending on what your hair needs and its individual characteristics, such as porosity and curl pattern.

It can be helpful to do a pre-conditioning process before we wash, to help coat the hair fibre to protect it from the washing process (known as hydra fatigue), as everything we do to our hair is a form of manipulation, which results in our hair strands becoming worn away as the hair becomes older.

Co-washing is a conditioning wash which is less drying than shampoos. However, this method should be used alongside a regimen of shampooing, as there is a risk of product build-up on the scalp and hair fibre, which could lead to scalp and hair problems. I normally recommend using a healthy shampoo each month if you are co-washing weekly or every two weeks.

Some healthy shampoos used by the Saffron Jade Family include: Aubrey Organics shampoo range and Camille Rose Naturals, Sweet Ginger Cleansing Rinse, Lena Maye Citrusy Herb Moisturising Shampoo (Website: lenamaye.co.uk). All are sulphate-free and have ingredients to nourish the hair and scalp.

Notes

Moisture Conditioners

Role is to increase the moisture content
of the hair and improve its elasticity.
Smooth the cuticle and soften
the hair fibre

The Purpose of Products
for Healthy Hair and Longer Lengths

Rinse-out Conditioners and Leave-in Conditioners

There are three main categories of conditioner, all which play an important part in the health and well-being of our hair. The focus in this section is:

- Rinse-out conditioners
- Leave-in conditioners.

A **daily or rinse-out conditioner** is a lightweight conditioner that can be used daily and is meant to be washed out (swimmers might need to wash their hair daily if swimming every day). This type of conditioner needs to have a lot of 'slip', meaning very slippery, as it helps to detangle our curls. You can use this before you wash your hair if your hair is very tangled or matted. However, be very gentle with your hair when it is wet, as it is most fragile then. This type of conditioner will hydrate your hair and helps it to be less frizzy as its purpose is to also smooth your cuticles and add softness. Think of when you add softener to your clothes after washing them.

Always use this type of conditioner when you get your hair wet and after you shampoo. The role of the conditioners is to refortify the cuticle with a protective coating and add additional moisture to the cortex, allowing the hair to keep growing without breaking.

A **leave-in conditioner** is to be used after washing your hair to replenish and maintain moisture. They are not rinsed out and are useful for controlling frizz and detangling strands and keeping curls smooth. These conditioners are normally light lotions, creams or liquids. Leave-in sprays are effective; they are easy to apply to the ends of their hair that need special attention and protection for retaining length.

A leave-in conditioner locks the moisture in the hair strands for a longer period than a conditioner you rinse out.

Healthy rinse-out conditioners include: Shea Moisture rinse-out conditioners, Giovanna Tea Tree Conditioner, Banana and Ginger rinse-out conditioners from The Body Shop, Aubrey Organics conditioners and the Aveda range, Lena Maye Citrusy Herb Moisturising Conditioner (Website: lenamaye.co.uk).

Leave-in conditioners: Shea Moisture Black Jamaican Castor Oil Leave-in Conditioner, Saffron Jade Rose Almond Leave-in Conditioning Moisture Spray, Alikay Naturals Lemongrass Leave-in Conditioner, Lena Maye Citrusy Herb Leave-in Conditioner. Other healthy brands include: Mielle Organics, TGIN and Afrocenchix.

Notes

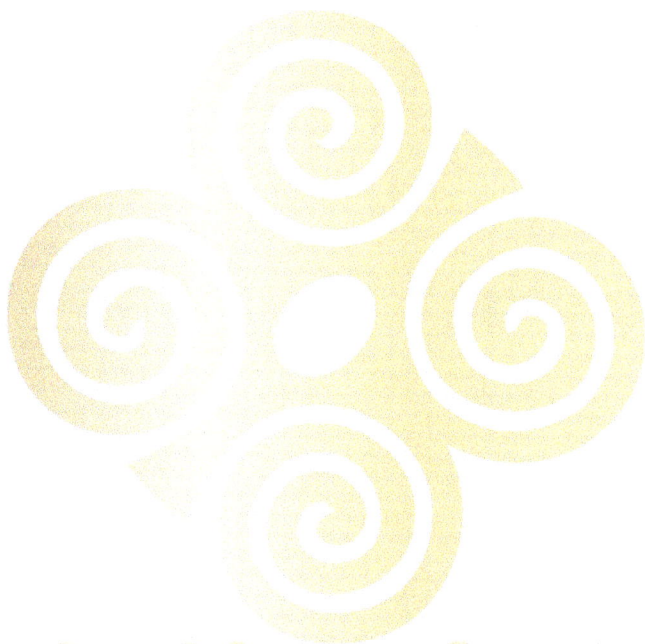

Protein Conditioners

Range from light to heavy concentration – role to strengthen and rebuild cuticle layer of hair fibre temporarily, (7 – 10 days) (4-6 weeks heavy protein treatments)

The Purpose of Products
for Healthy Hair and Longer Lengths

Protein Conditioner

Our hair is made up of a protein called keratin, which makes up approximately 91% of the strand. When our hair lacks protein, it's essentially missing its DNA. This affects the strength and resilience of the hair strand to be able to withstand the day-to-day manipulation of combing, washing, styling etc. If protein is lost and not replaced, the hair will become weak and eventually break off. Other things that affect the protein structure of the hair include:

- Chemicals, including dyes, weakening the hair structure

- Poor care, leading to cuticle damage

- A poor diet lacking in protein foods.

Light protein conditioners and deep conditioners that are protein based can be used weekly or fortnightly as part of a healthy haircare regimen to support a moisture / protein balance depending on your individual hair needs. Reconstructors and protein packs are generally designed for more damaged hair and are recommended to be used monthly, depending on the hair's health and the needs of the individual.

What might indicate that my hair needs a protein treatment?

- Hair feels soft and mushy and unable to hold a curl, or appears stringy
- When you stretch your hair, it breaks off
- Hair appears limp and lifeless.

Some protein conditioners used by the Saffron Jade family: ApHogee Keratin 2-Minute Reconstructor (light protein), Giovanni Reconstructor, Aveda Rescue Remedy.

Notes

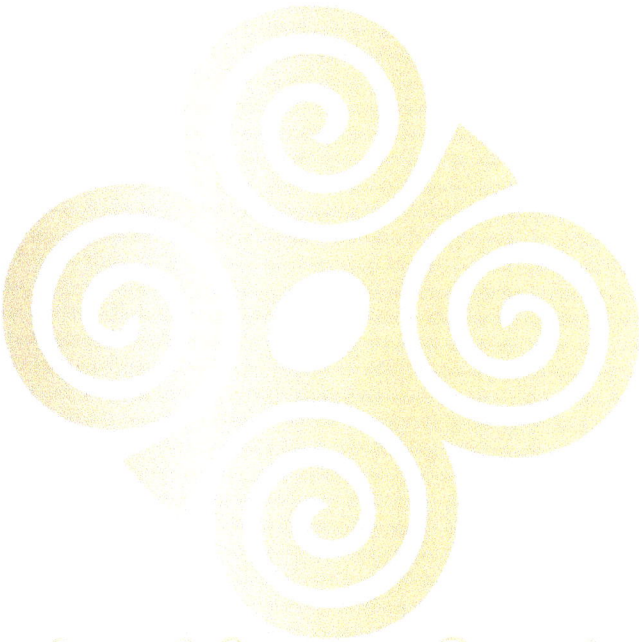

Deep Conditioners & Treatments

Adds essential ingredients which penetrate the hair shaft

The Purpose of Products
for Healthy Hair and Longer Lengths

Deep Conditioning

A **deep conditioner** is an intensive moisturising and nourishing treatment, also called 'deep treatment' and 'masque'. These can be broken down into two categories: those meant to provide proteins and those primarily for moisture. As we know, healthy hair is a balance between moisture and protein, so we need to use both, depending on the individual needs of our hair. These conditioners are normally quite thick in consistency and should be left on the hair, with heat, for 20-30 minutes. Think of deep conditioners as a five-star meal for your hair. This type of treatment has significant benefits to the overall health and well-being of Afro-textured hair.

Deep treatments can be used weekly or fortnightly depending on the current health status of your hair and individual needs.

Some of the deep treatments used by Saffron Jade family are brands such as: Shea Moisture range of deep treatments, Giovanni range of deep treatments, Aubrey Organics deep treatments and Aveda treatments. Other healthy brands include: Mielle Organics, TGIN and Afrocenchix.

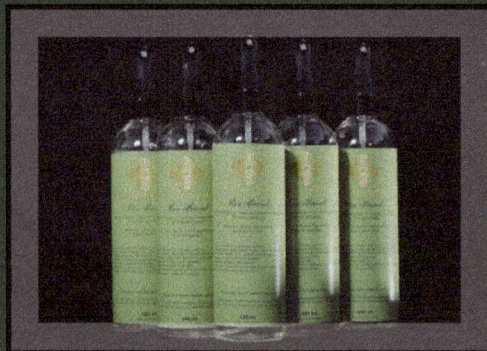

The Purpose of Products
for Healthy Hair and Longer Lengths

Saffron Jade.
Rose Almond – Natural Organic Leave-in
Conditioning Moisture Spray for Hair and Scalp

Saffron Jade's Rose Almond 'Natural Organic Leave-in Conditioning Moisture spray for hair and scalp was formulated to provide customers with curly, coily Afro-textured hair with leave-in conditioning moisture spray for healthy hair, whilst promoting a healthy scalp. The use of the spray has several benefits, with the main function being to keep hair hydrated to support a healthy pH balance, adding essential moisture, promoting elasticity and natural shine.

The spray's formulation is designed for Afro-textured hair and the need to add additional moisture, through a regimen of regular hydration and essential oils for optimum hair growth. This can also be used for natural or relaxed hair. Furthermore, it is essential for hair in weaves or braid extensions to be maintained with a regimen of regular hydration and moisture. When sprayed daily or every other day, hair will maintain a healthy level of moisture to remain hydrated and soft to prevent dryness, which leads to breakage.

Naturally active ingredients include aloe vera and vitamin E, natural conditioners for the hair and scalp to promote healthy hair growth, almond oil to increase lustre and shine. Carrot seed and rosemary stimulate hair growth, whilst supporting longer and stronger hair.

Rose Almond Leave-in Conditioning Spray can be used as part of a two-phase process, for wet or dry hair, and / or as a heat protector for blow-drying.

Phase one: Section hair and spray sections, working product through from root to tip.

Phase two: Depending on the thickness of the hair and porosity: after working product from root to tip, seal with a moisture cream, shea butter or curling cream to prolong hydration and moisture retention of the hair.

For hair weaves: Spray scalp and root of hair, to add essential moisture to prevent dryness and breakage for the duration of the weave hairstyle.

For braid extensions: Spray scalp, root of hair and the braid to where the hair ends, to add essential moisture to prevent dryness and breakage for the duration of the braid hairstyle.

For Locs: Depending on the hair's ability to retain moisture: after working product from root to tip, seal with additional pure oil of choice, e.g: olive oil, coconut oil to prolong hydration and moisture retention of the hair.

Heat Protector: Section hair in four to six sections, or for individual rollers. Spray each section from root to tip, paying extra attention to the ends of the hair before blow-drying or rolling, using a moderate heat.

Notes

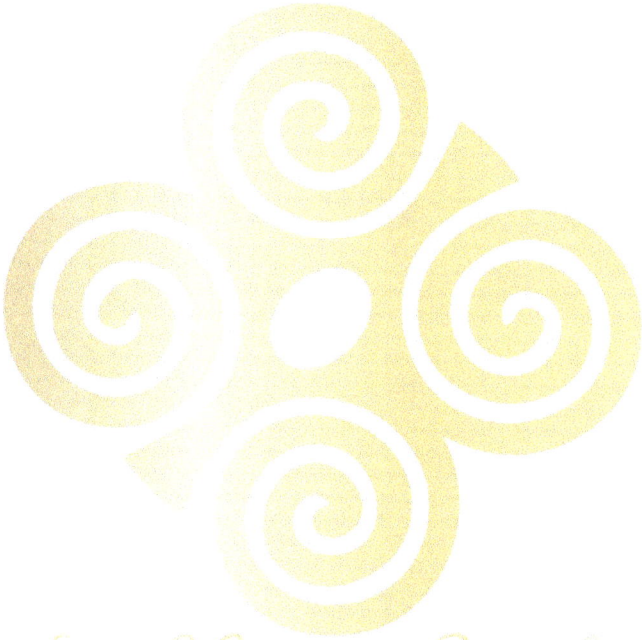

Creams & Gels

- ✤ **BUTTER CREAMS**

- ✤ **CURLING CREAMS**

- ✤ **GELS**

The Purpose of Products
for Healthy Hair and Longer Lengths

Creams / Gels

The role of a moisturising or curling cream is to both condition and moisturise our hair, helping it feel soft and flexible, allowing our curls to bounce and shine. The nature of the ingredients will affect how well it does this, as we already spoke about seeing products as food for the hair. A moisture cream needs to have water as a key ingredient, to add moisture to our hair. A good curl cream will also enhance the natural pattern of our hair by encouraging curl formation, allowing them to be the best version of themselves.

Gels are used to style our hair and give us additional hold, depending on the style and look we are trying to achieve. Gels provide a longer-lasting wash-and-go by sealing moisture underneath and controlling frizz for a defined curl. A healthy gel can define your curls without leaving them feeling dry and flaky.

When to use them?

A moisturising gel will be unable to provide as much moisture as a cream, which is why many women like myself use a cream and then a gel, to get the best of both worlds. This allows me to use a cream to moisturise my hair and a gel to ensure it has a good hold and shine throughout the day, whilst I am at work. I then use my Saffron Jade Natural Leave-in Moisture Spray daily to keep my hair with a good balance of moisture, adding a healthy gel daily for hold, until my wash day.

Some of the creams and gels used by the Saffron Jade family: Aloe Vera Gel, Dr Organics from Holland and Barrett; Alikay Naturals SHEA YOGURT Hair Moisturiser; Design Essentials Almond & Avocado Curl Stretching Cream; tgin Butter Cream Daily Moisturizer; Eden Bodyworks Coco-Shea Berry Smoothing Gel.

Notes

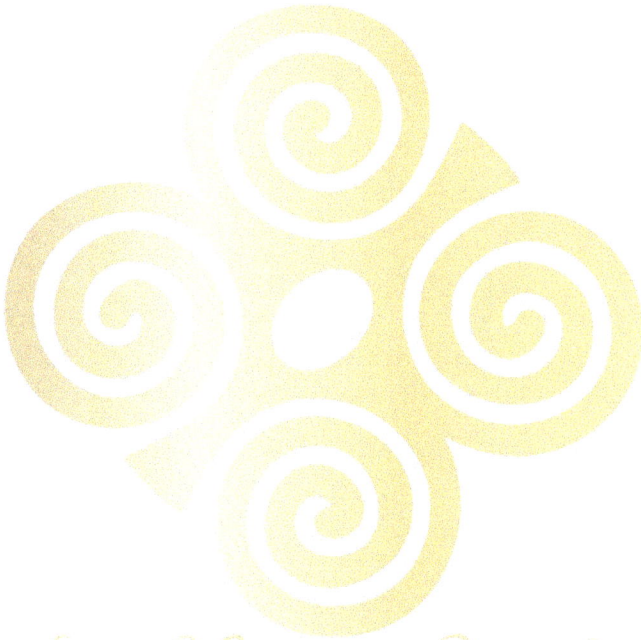

LOC / LCO Method

Liquid, Oil and Cream
for prolonged hydration
and moisture retention

The Purpose of Products for Healthy Hair and Longer Lengths

LOC / LCO Method

What is the Liquid Oil Cream or Liquid Cream and Oil Method or LOC/LCO and how does it work?

The Liquid Oil Cream Method, or LOC method, is a technique for moisturising hair. The LCO method, Liquid Cream and Oil, is a slight variation, with the cream being applied before the oil. Rochelle Alikay Graham-Campbell of Alikay Naturals credits herself for coining the term and trademarking it.

The method consists of hydrating the hair with water or a water-based product, which is your liquid, sealing in the moisture with oil and then applying a cream product to close the hair cuticle, which prevents moisture loss.

The LOC Method or Liquid Oil Cream Method is a guide for how to apply your products to ensure your hair is moisturised and stays moisturised longer, which is essential for Afro-textured hair. The method works for:

- Naturally curly hair
- Relaxed hair
- Locs.

Three reasons the LOC method works:

1. Water represents moisture – which is essential for our health in the short and longer term.

2. Oil ensures the hair holds on to the water – it's best to use an oil that is pure and can penetrate the hair shaft to enter the cortex of the hair, such as coconut, olive and avocado oil, castor oil, jojoba oil, almond oil, etc.

3. Cream or a product that seals in the moisture. The purpose of the cream is to seal or lock in moisture introduced from liquid and oil. Oils that seal include castor oil, grapeseed and jojoba. Some of these oils can also act as emollients that lubricate and fill in gaps along the hair cuticle to prevent moisture loss.

This is a method which provides great benefits to keeping the hair hydrated for a longer period; natural, relaxed or wearing beautiful locs. If you have locs and do not like using a cream, as some cause build-up, you can seal with just the oil.

(naturalhairrules.com/loc-method/)

Notes

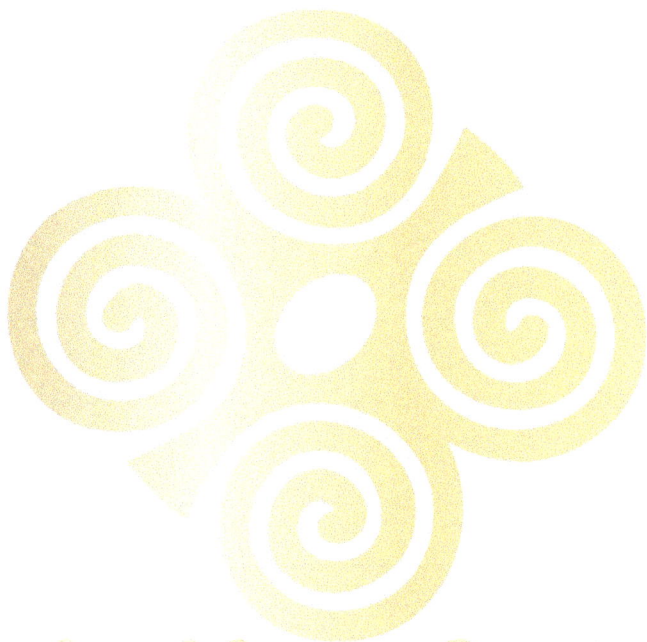

Healthy Hair Tools

Finger de-tangling, wide
tooth combs, Denman brush,
hair bands, soft brushes
to smooth cuticle

The Purpose of Products
for Healthy Hair and Longer Lengths

Healthy Hair Tools

Our hair loves to party and mingle, and our curls can become easily tangled. To keep our hair free from knots and tangles, we need to be extra careful in the way we manage our hair, to preserve it from the damage of everyday living, also known as weathering.

Understanding the damage tools can cause to our hair is essential when adopting your own individual healthy haircare regimen. These tools help to secure our hair, smooth, curl, stretch and comb it, but we need to ensure they do not damage our hair whilst we are using them. Some tips:

- The use of our hands is a great way to protect our hair, through finger detangling before washing and restyling

- Take extra care to avoid breaking hair when using combs

- Combing and brushing – be gentle, so as not to strip the cuticle layer and cause damage

- Style with bands and clips, accessories that do not have metal that can tear the hair

- Protect our hair at night with a satin scarf whilst we sleep.

Your
Healthy Hair
Care Regimen

Getting Started
1. Commit
2. Assess & Plan
3. Products
4. Begin
5. Enjoy

COMMIT

PLAN

PRODUCTS

BEGIN

ENJOY

CHAPTER 8

Healthy Haircare Regimen

What do we mean when we talk about a healthy haircare regimen?

Healthy haircare means the care and attention that is given to ensuring our hair's best health. Saffron Jade promotes a holistic approach to healthy haircare, recognising the importance of adopting a healthy lifestyle of mind, body and spirit.

A regimen is a routine and a way of doing things consistently, like other routines, that gives positive results, such as doing physical activity three times a week. Adopting a regimen provides structure, repetition and consistency, so that taking care of your hair becomes a normal part of your everyday life.

I use my weekly cleanse/conditioning regimen time for self-reflection, time with myself, which supports my emotional, mental and spiritual well-being.

My wash day songs by Kirk Franklin include: *Hello Fear, Just for Me, Imagine Me, I Smile, Love Theory, 123 Victory, September* (album version) and *You Are. Chronixx I Can.*

Commit

Make a commitment to yourself
to dedicate the time and space
for a healthy hair regimen and
getting to know and understand
the characteristics of your hair

Healthy Haircare Regimen

Commit

Your hair is a special part of you – and you are one. Your commitment to developing a healthy relationship with your hair, getting to know and understand it and making the time to give it the respect, love and care that it requires is making a commitment to yourself. This commitment will include:

- Getting to know and understand your hair, realising this takes time, so patience is key

- Riding through rocky times; developing new relationships is never smooth

- Making the time and space to care for your hair a priority. This might include doing less for others, so you have more time for yourself.

- Becoming the expert of your hair, so you can understand how to meet its needs, as this can change for several reasons.

Assess & Plan

- Assess the current health of your hair

- Review your current regimen against what you have learned

- Set goals for your hair

- Plan a consistent regimen that will work for your lifestyle

NATURAL HAIR

RELAXED HAIR

CHILDREN'S HAIR

LOCS

BRAIDS

WEAVES

Healthy Haircare Regimen

Assess and Plan

The assessment of your hair's overall health will need to take into account its characteristics, such as texture (fine, medium or thick strands), your porosity, elasticity and the strength of your hair. The assessment of your hair should also include:

1. Damage or hair loss, such as breakage, thinning at the edges and the amount of heat you use on your hair.

2. The current weathering of your hair, based on the age of your hair fibres and how well they have been cared for. Are your strands damaged?

3. Your weekly regimen of activity, gym, swimming, and the need to cleanse more often.

4. Do you have chemically treated hair, including dye?

5. A timescale for your regimen – whether it's weekly, fortnightly, every three weeks or two or three times a week

6. Does your hair need a daily routine for moisturising?

7. Remember, your assessment is ongoing, as changes to your life and lifestyle are constant and will have an impact on your hair. These changes can include age, physical health, changes in your environment, etc.

All this will help you think about the products and possible changes in styling your hair that best support its health needs.

The planning of a regimen will need to factor in all the things below, after assessing your individual hair. Not everything will apply to everyone but, at a basic level, the ones highlighted with an asterisk should form part of a consistent regimen.

- Pre-conditioning
- Detangling process*
- Cleansing/shampoo*
- Protein conditioning*
- Moisturising conditioning*
- Deep conditioning*
- LOC/LCO – liquid, oils, creams
- Moisture cream or spray*
- Heat protector
- Low manipulation and protective styling
- Protecting hair at night – silk scarf/pillowcase

Case Examples of Healthy Haircare Regimens

Lauren is 45 years old and has had her locs for eight years. She has low-density hair and her hair texture is fine, with medium porosity. She likes to attend her appointment with her loctician once every six to eight weeks, when she gets her hair washed, conditioned and styled. Lauren was experiencing itchy scalp and some dandruff and was concerned about her locs feeling dry and brittle. She decided to adopt a healthier haircare regimen.

Lauren's new healthy haircare regimen is as follows:

- Changed to using an organic shampoo, sulphate-free
- Washing and conditioning her locs in between her visit to get her hair retwisted
- Pre-conditioning with coconut oil
- Light protein treatment every three weeks, to keep locs strong and healthy
- Using a rinse-out moisturising conditioner – she leaves this in her hair for 20-30 minutes, to allow the product to fully penetrate its cortex, helping her locs to be fully hydrated and add softness
- Deep conditioning with a heat every three weeks, as Lauren dyes her hair
- Use of Saffron Jade Moisture Spray every other day to keep locs topped up with a good level of moisture. She seals with a natural oil.
- Ensuring her locs are not twisted too often or too tightly.

Jade has had her relaxed since she was 16 years old and is now 25. Her hair texture is medium, and she has high-porosity hair, which is largely due to the chemical use of the relaxer. She had been washing her hair every four to six weeks and would follow up with a conditioner, only leaving it in her hair for a few minutes. She has been experiencing breakage at the back and sides. She sometimes blow-dries her hair without using a heat protector.

Jade's new weekly healthy haircare regimen is as follows:

- Pre-conditioning with coconut oil – leave in for 20 minutes if possible

- Shampoo with sulphate-free – wash hair in four to six sections of loose twist/braids to avoid hair becoming tangled

- Use of a light to medium protein conditioner (leave in for 20-30 minutes)

- Moisture conditioner – 30 minutes

- Deep treatment – moisture base for 30 minutes with heat

- Leave-in conditioner, and LOC method, before styling

- Sprays hair with Saffron Jade Moisture Spray at night before she wraps her hair and sleeps with her silk scarf, paying attention to the ends of her hair

- Jade's protective hairstyle for three months: She will be wearing her hair in a bun with ends tucked away to support length retention.

Sharon is 32 and has natural hair, of very fine texture and medium porosity. She has a medium density and eats a balanced diet. Sharon had been washing her hair weekly and conditioning but was only leaving the conditioner on for five minutes. She was not always deep conditioning and not using any protein conditioners within her regimen. She was able to see her beautiful natural curl pattern being consistent with her weekly regimen, but she wanted her curls more defined and felt her hair could be more resilient. Sharon's preferred style of choice is a wash-and-go.

Sharon's new weekly healthy haircare regimen:

- Detangling her hair gently with her fingers, to ensure no knots or tangles in preparation for washing

- Pre-conditioning with coconut oil or olive oil

- Shampoo with sulphate-free – wash hair in four to six sections of loose twist/braids to avoid hair becoming tangled

- Use of a light to medium protein conditioner (leave in for 20 minutes)

- Moisture conditioner for 30 minutes

- Deep treatment – moisture base for 30 minutes with heat

- Leave-in conditioner, and LOC method before styling, using curling cream and gel for more defined curls

- Sprays hair with Saffron Jade Moisture Spray at night before she wraps her hair and sleeps with her silk scarf

- Sharon just fluffs up her wash-and-go with a pick comb in the morning. Hair remains untouched until the wash day regimen. This supports greater length retention.

Pauline is 17 and has natural hair which she likes to wear in extension braids. She has thick textured hair and medium porosity. Before she started her healthy haircare regimen, she used to keep her braids in for around six to eight weeks, or sometimes longer. Her care of her hair whilst in these braids was minimal, although she did ensure her edges were not braided and the braids were not too tight. She understood that her hair follicles could become permanently damaged and result in hair loss.

Pauline did not have a consistent regimen when her hair was not in braids. Her hair was constantly dry, and she would experience a lot of breakage when she removed her braids. She was unable to see her natural curl pattern, due to the deficiency of moisture within her hair cortex.

Pauline's New Healthy Haircare Regimen:

- Pauline leaves her braids in for a minimum of six weeks, and washes and conditions her hair whilst in the braids every two to three weeks

- She sprays her hair whilst in the braids every other day, to where her hair ends and the roots, with Saffron Jade Moisture Spray

- Once she takes them out of the braids, she does a full routine of wash, conditioning, light protein conditioning and deep conditioning

- She gives her hair a break from the tension of the braids for three weeks and ensures she does a full healthy haircare routine before she puts her braids back.

Children's Healthy Haircare Regimen:

It is essential we set an example of a healthy haircare regimen for children from an early age, considering all the learning we have covered within this masterclass. This will help children to not only become experts of their hair as they grow, but it will also mean that their hair looks and feels healthy, allowing them to see their naturally beautiful curly hair as a normal part of their cultural identity. This supports self-love, self-acceptance and self-confidence from an early age, which is important for positive mental and emotional well-being.

0-two years: Haircare for new-born's and toddlers should be kept very simple, as the hair is very fine due to the hair fibres being in the early stages of developing and changing. For some children, this early stage will continue until the age of three, as each child is different. As children grow, their texture will begin to pick up. At this stage, children's hair can be rinsed with warm water, as shampoos are not said to be necessary. You can use a light conditioner as the hair becomes thicker in texture. A light natural oil, such as olive oil, should be enough whilst children have the fine hair textures. As the hair becomes thicker, a light moisturising cream, followed by a light oil to retain the moisture, can be used.

Three years and above: Once children's hair texture matures and hair thickens, the hair fibre will need care the same as for your hair. The slight differences will be that children's hair is rarely damaged, so they will not need protein conditioners, probably until they reach 11 years-plus. All the products used on children's hair should support the need for our hair to have moisture. Shampoos and conditioners should be sulphate-free and creamy and rich. This is the time when children's hair should be in a protective hair style braids with their own hair as much as possible for school, as low-manipulation styles will ensure they retain their length. Non-braided hair can be worn on the weekend, after braids are taken out, ready for weekly washing and conditioning. The move away from children's hair being mostly braided from two to 11-years-old is costing them their length and the general health of the hair, due to it being manipulated daily.

Many children are having their hair damaged in a number of ways, which will lead to hair problems as they get older. It is our responsibility as parents/carers to protect them from this damage. See information and tips below about keeping children's hair healthy.

- Children's scalps are very sensitive and delicate. It is not advised for children under seven years to have braid extensions, due to the weight and tension caused to the scalp.

- Braids that are too tight can damage the hair follicle, leading to hair loss

- Braid extensions being left in too long, without the hair being washed and conditioned. You can wash and condition children's hair weekly whilst in braids.

- Weekly or fortnightly regimen of washing and conditioning. Scalps need to be clean for hair to grow healthy.

- Hair needs to be moisturised during the week to keep it from drying out and breaking. This will be different for each child, depending on hair porosity, texture and curl pattern.

- Unhealthy shampoos and conditioners being used that strip the hair of essential moisture.

Products
& Styling

Select your healthy products — based on the needs of Afro-textured hair and your unique characteristics as discussed earlier.

Remember your goal is to strike the right moisture / protein balance, low manipulation and protective styling.

Healthy Haircare Regimen

Selecting Your Individual Products and Styling Plan

The selection of your products and styling plan should be based around your individual hair needs. You should be constantly assessing your hair for changes, as the needs will alter depending on your lifestyle, environment, health and the care or lack of care you have been providing for your hair.

What products should you be thinking of and what styling options should you be thinking about?

- Cleansing/shampoo
- Conditioning – balance between moisture and protein
- What type of ingredients work for the characteristics of your hair? Use the case studies as an example to guide your thinking about your own hair and goals.
- Deep conditioning – heat cap/steamer
- What oils work best for your hair? How are you going to use your oils?
- Do you need a styling cream/gel for your preferred style?
- If your goal is to achieve longer lengths alongside the health of your hair, what protective styles will you adopt?
- If you are experiencing hair loss/damage due to the styling of your hair, you need to change this practice to allow your hair to grow back
- Don't forgot your silk scarf/bonnet at night to protect your hair.

Begin

Begin your regimen, set a time
of 6 – 12 weeks
to review your progress.

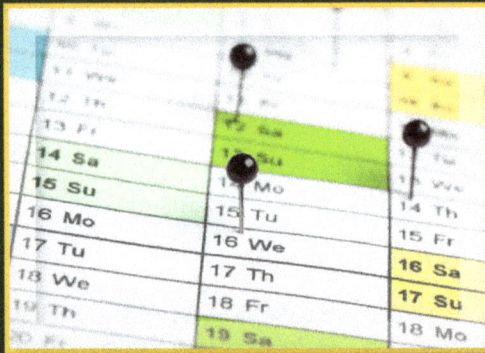

Enjoy

Enjoy the journey, have patience
as getting to know and understand
your unique hair takes time.

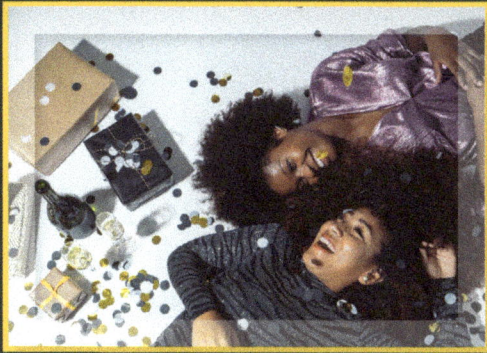

Notes

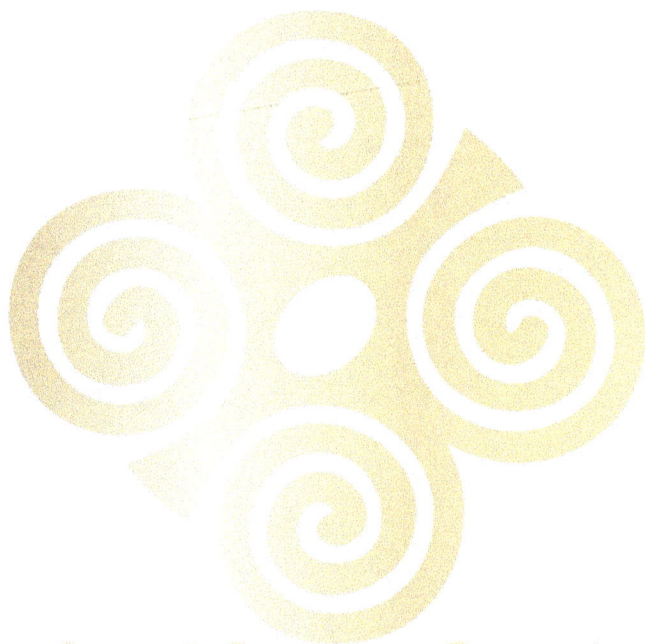

Begin and Enjoy

Your beginning will be individual to you and your hair. It will be your own starting point. It does not matter whether this is your first time beginning your journey to investing in the health of your hair or are at the start of a new beginning. If you stop at any point, you only need to choose to begin again.

Once you begin your healthy haircare regimen, pencil in a review date of six to twelve weeks. It's important to review your progress so you can decide if any part of your regimen needs changes. You can then review every three months as your journey continues.

Most importantly, enjoy the journey of getting to know and understand your hair, and know that you are not alone, as we are all on this beautiful journey together.

Acknowledgements

We can do all things 'by He who gives us strength' Firstly, I would like to thank our Higher Being for the love and guidance I have always felt in supporting me to keep going and remain positive and thankful throughout the difficulties and challenges we all face in everyday life. I am also thankful to my family and close friends for the love, support and encouragement I continue to receive. Your belief in me has enabled me to continue to pursue my goals and passion.

Lastly, a message to my black and mixed heritage Saffron Jade family all over the world, and especially those who have encouraged me to keep going with my passion for education on healthy hair within our community. Your intelligence, strength, courage, resilience, creativity and beauty make you all truly amazing.

This book is dedicated to all my black and mixed heritage Saffron Jade family, celebrating you and your hair.

Special thanks to Conscious Dreams Publishing team: Lee Dickinson editor, Nadia Vitushynska typesetter and Daniella Blechner, Book Journey Mentor and Publisher for making my book a reality.

References

Books

Angela Adams McGhee (2015). *Definitive Trichology's Complete Guide to Healthy, Beautiful Hair.*

Chicoro (2009). *Grow It: How To Grow Afro-Textured Hair to Maximum Lengths in the Shortest Time.*

Audrey Davis-Sivasothy (2011). *The Science of Black Hair – A Comprehensive Guide to Textured Hair Care, 2011.*

Websites

www.boucleme.co.uk/blogs/news/the-difference-between-curl-cream-vs-curl-defining-gel

www.naturallycurly.com/texture-typing/density

www.cosmopolitan.com/uk/beauty-hair/advice/a48958/hair-loss-reasons/

www.hairfinder.com/hairquestions/hairelasticity

www.curlsandpotions.com

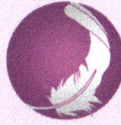

Conscious Dreams
P U B L I S H I N G

Be the author of your own destiny

Find out about our authors, events, services
and how you too can get your book journey started.

Conscious Dreams Publishing

@DreamsConscious

@consciousdreamspublishing

Daniella Blechner

www.consciousdreamspublishing.com

info@consciousdreamspublishing.com

Let's connect

www.ingramcontent.com/pod-product-compliance
Lightning Source LLC
Chambersburg PA
CBHW042248040426
42336CB00043B/3363